Up to the Sky,
Around the World &
Deep in My Heart

by Janelle Basham

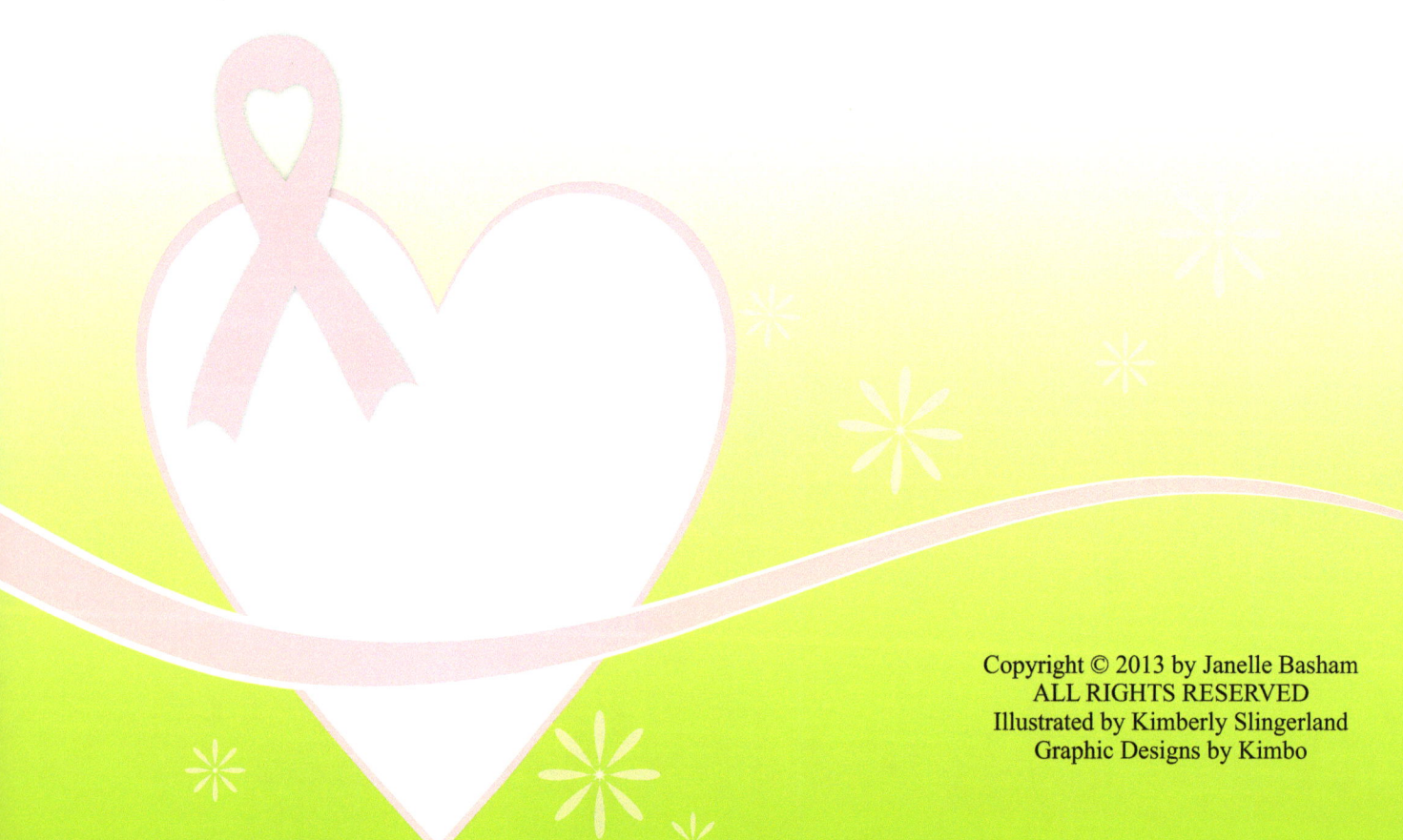

This book is dedicated to my mother Celene, my children Jocelyn, Kaitlyn & Kyle and all the courageous children of breast cancer survivors.

Copyright © 2013 by Janelle Basham
ALL RIGHTS RESERVED
Illustrated by Kimberly Slingerland
Graphic Designs by Kimbo

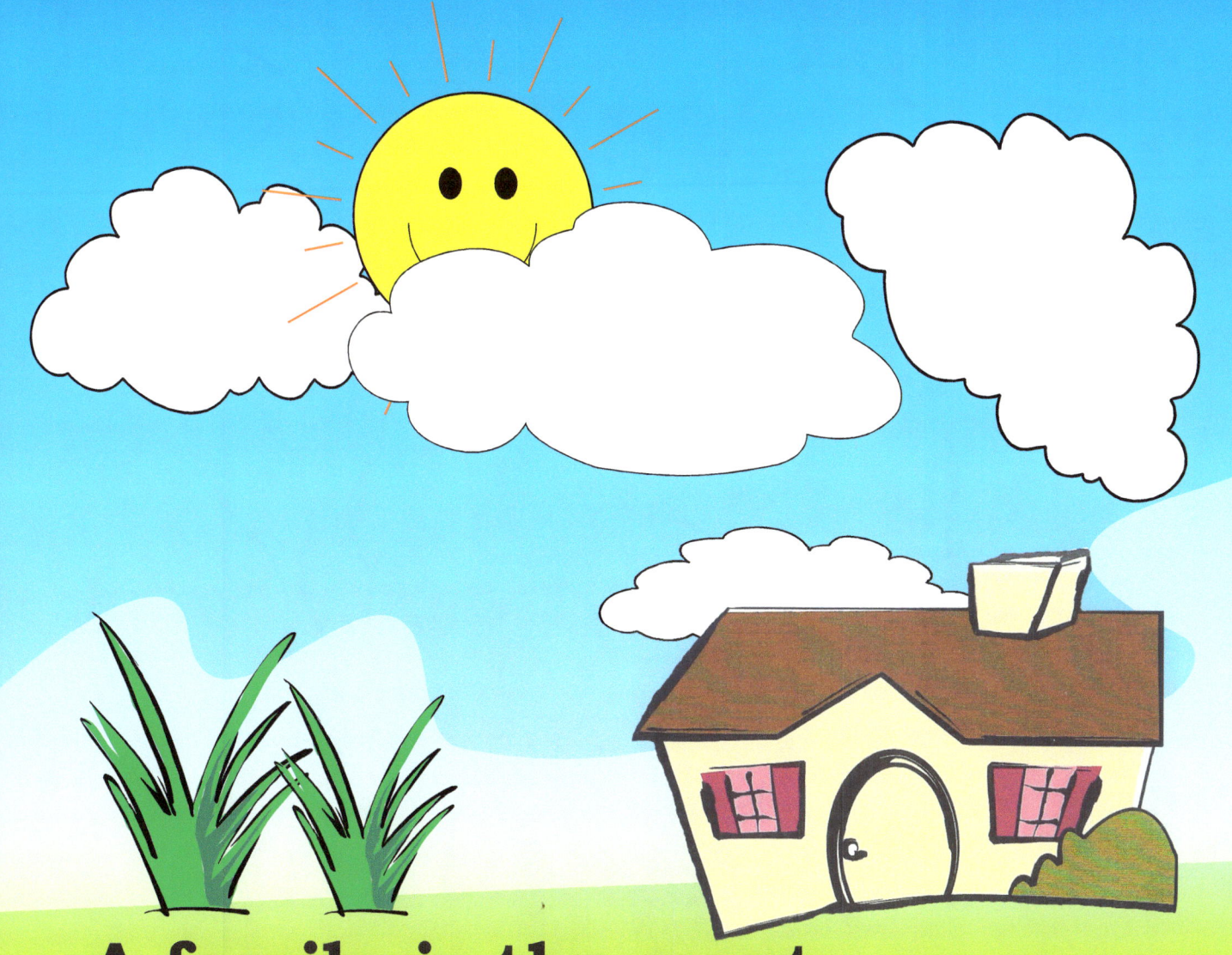

A family is the most important gift little boys and girls will have in their whole entire lives. Even longer!

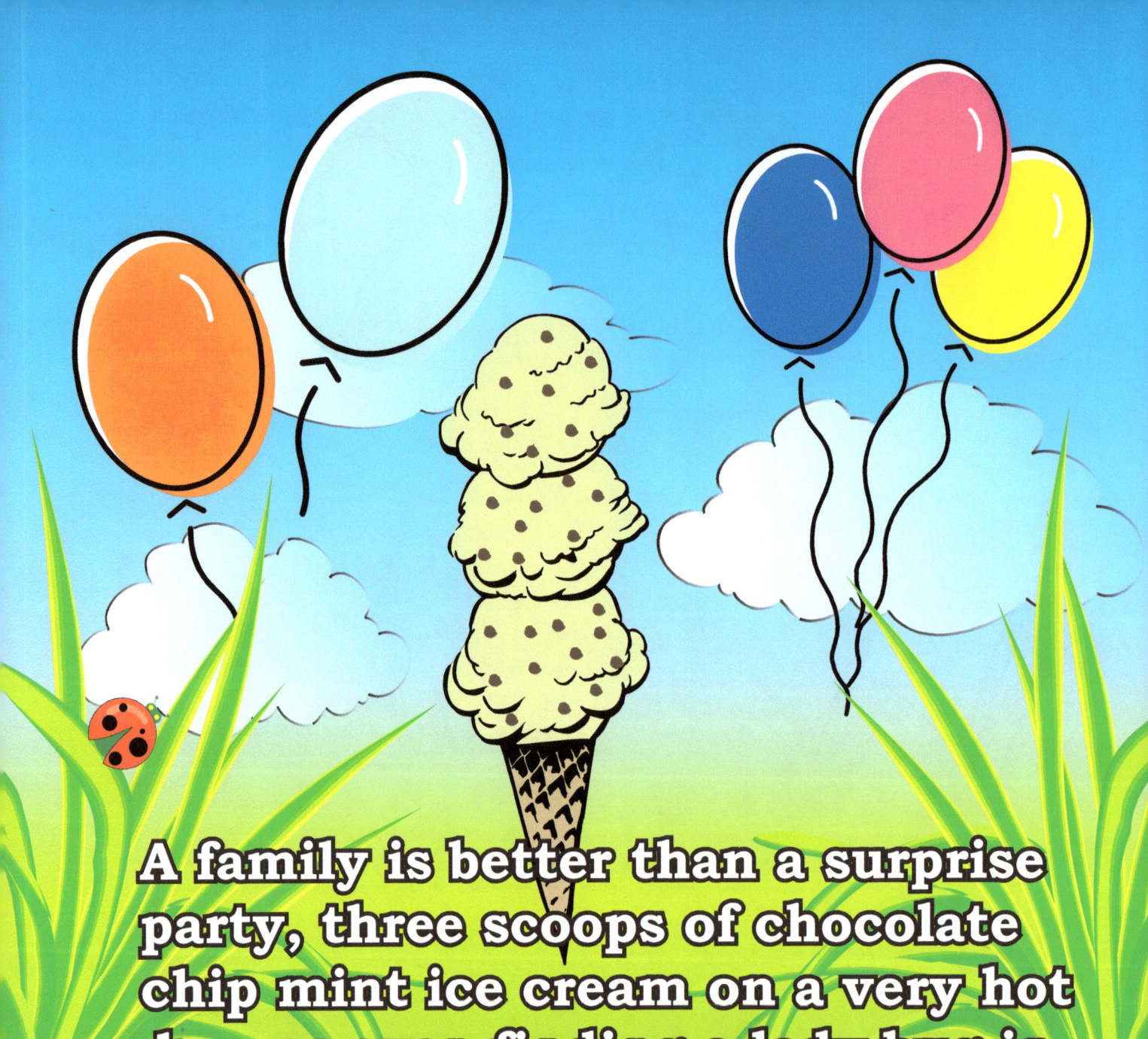

A family is better than a surprise party, three scoops of chocolate chip mint ice cream on a very hot day, or even finding a lady bug in the tall green grass.

Families are always there to lean on. They support and celebrate all that each other does. Whether it is an amazing dance competition, or eating all your broccoli.

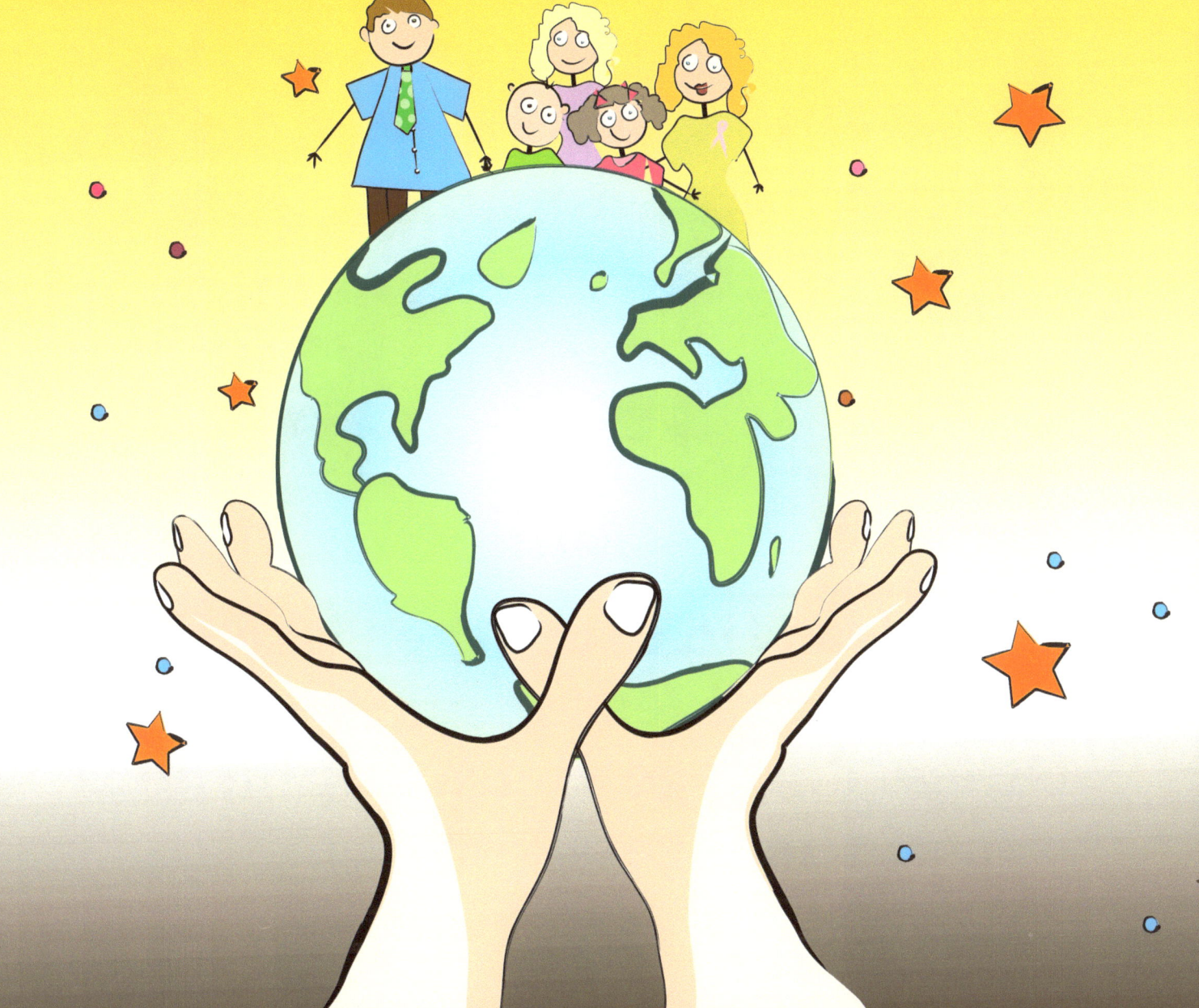

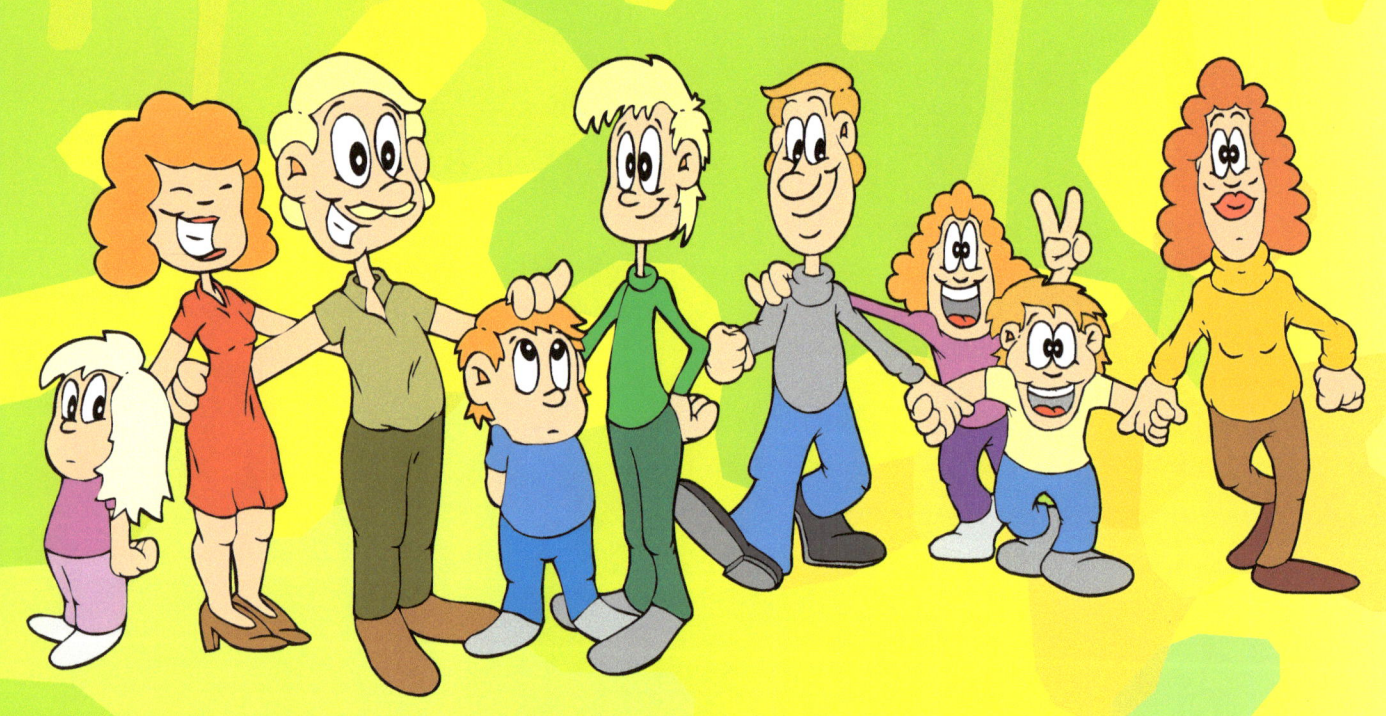

Families stick together like the world's stickiest glue; even when things don't go right. Like when one of them gets sick.

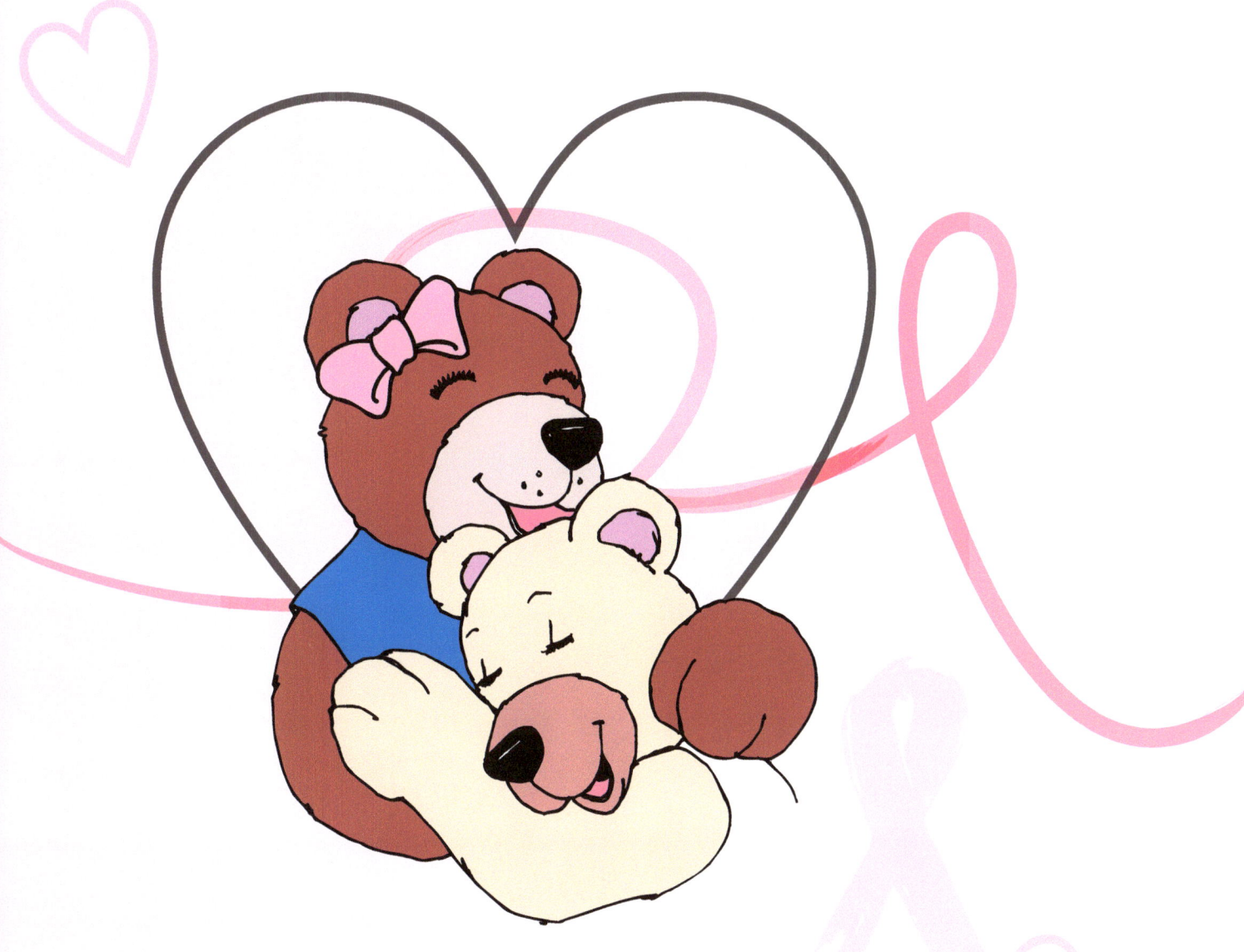

Deep inside where you cannot see is where Mommy is sick. It is called Breast Cancer.

The cells in mommy's breast are sick. It is not like a cold that you can catch. Most women don't even know they have breast cancer until a doctor tells them.

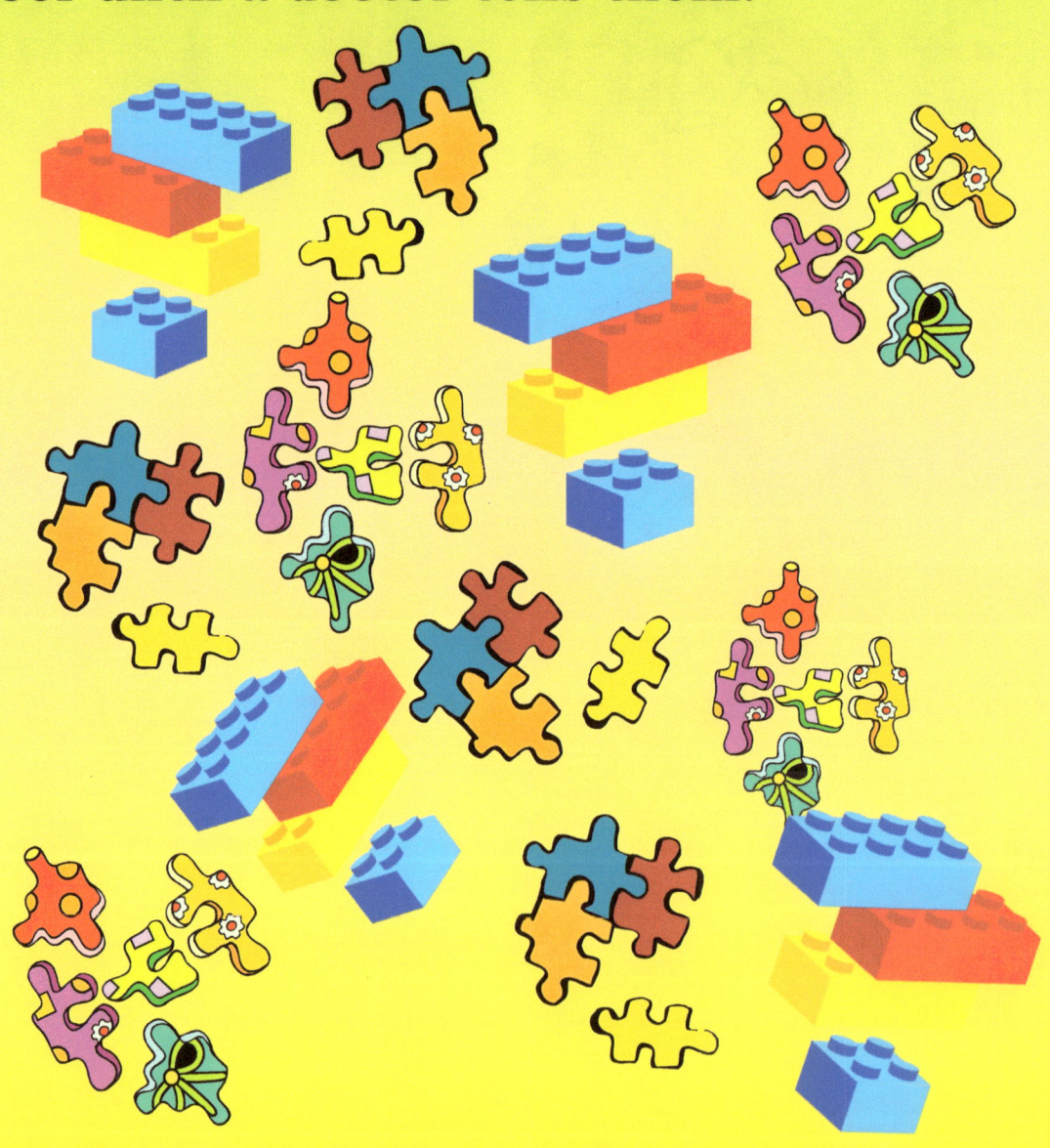

Millions and millions of tiny little round things called CELLS make up our body. The cells work very hard to keep the body working in tip top shape. They work like building blocks.

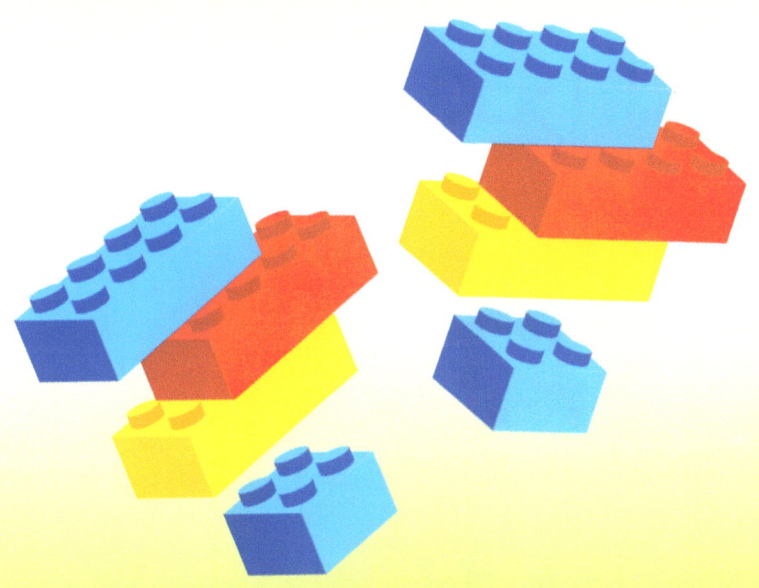

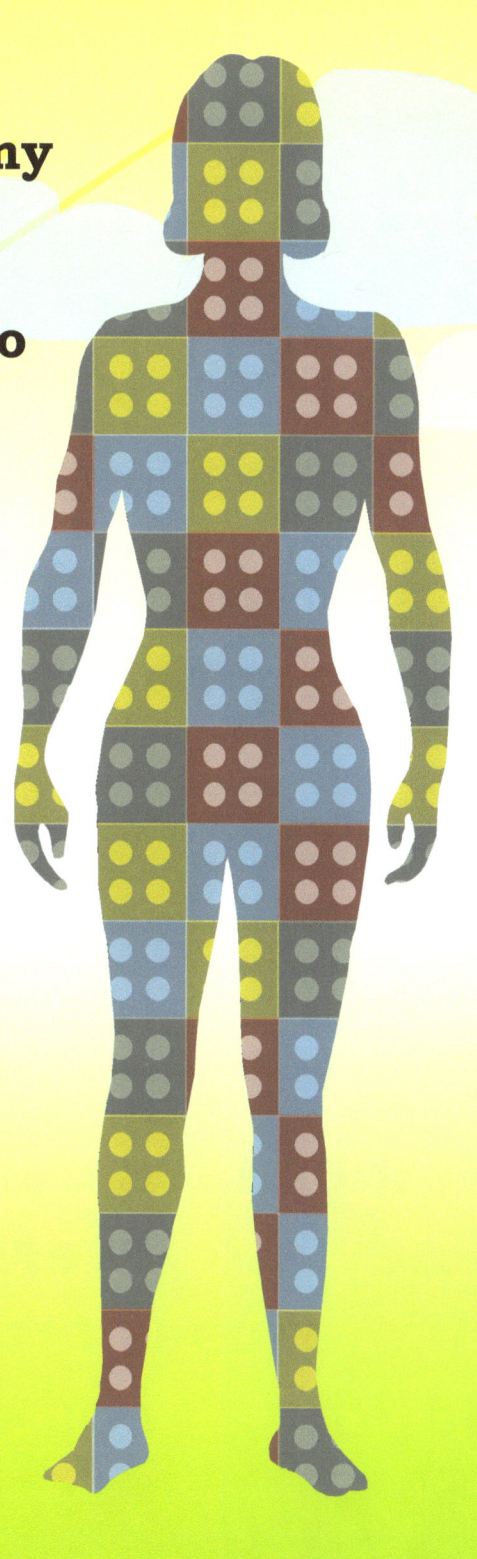

Each day they attach to each other and build a strong, healthy body.

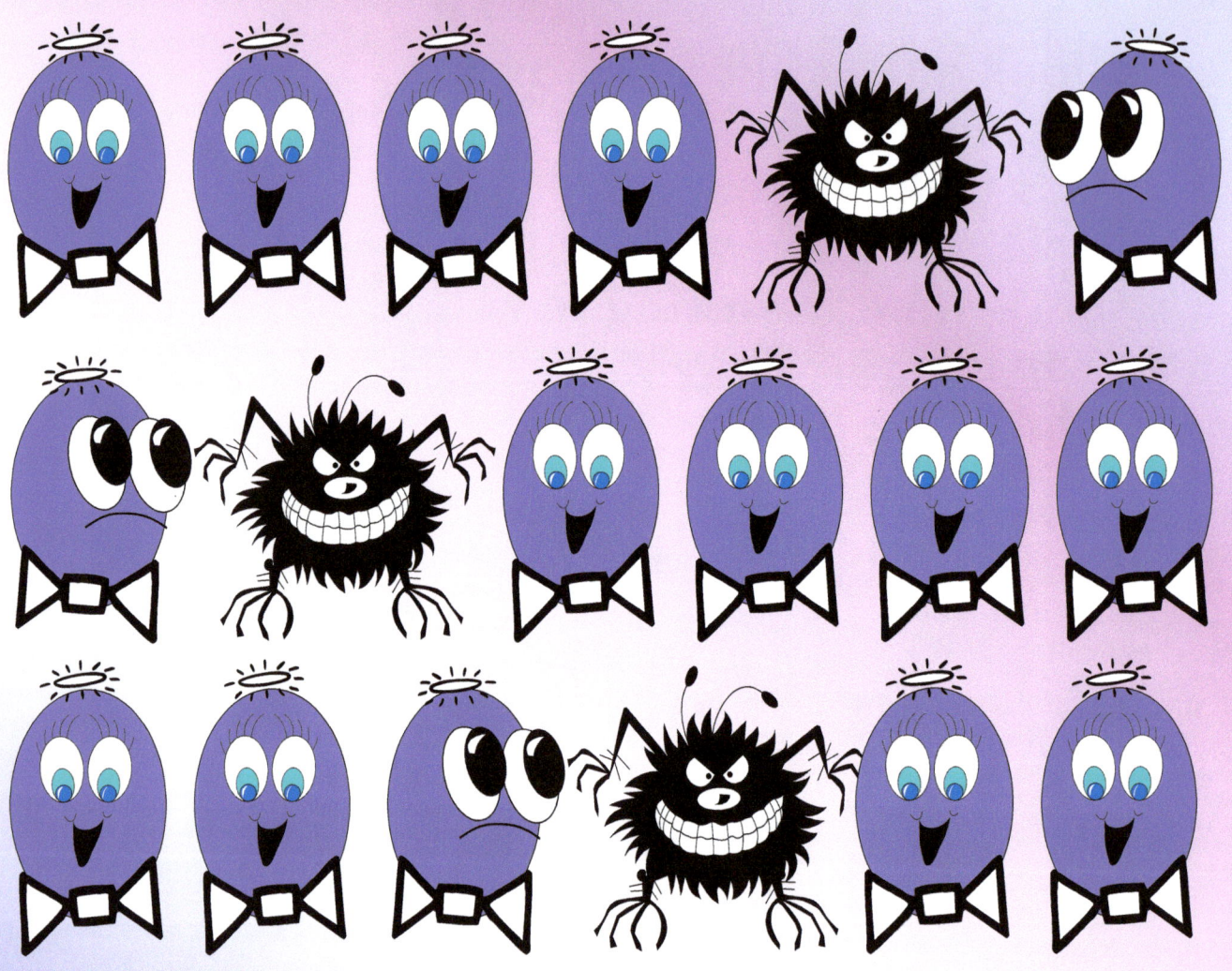

Sometimes cells get a bad attitude. They stop working together and this causes trouble. The body stops building good cells.

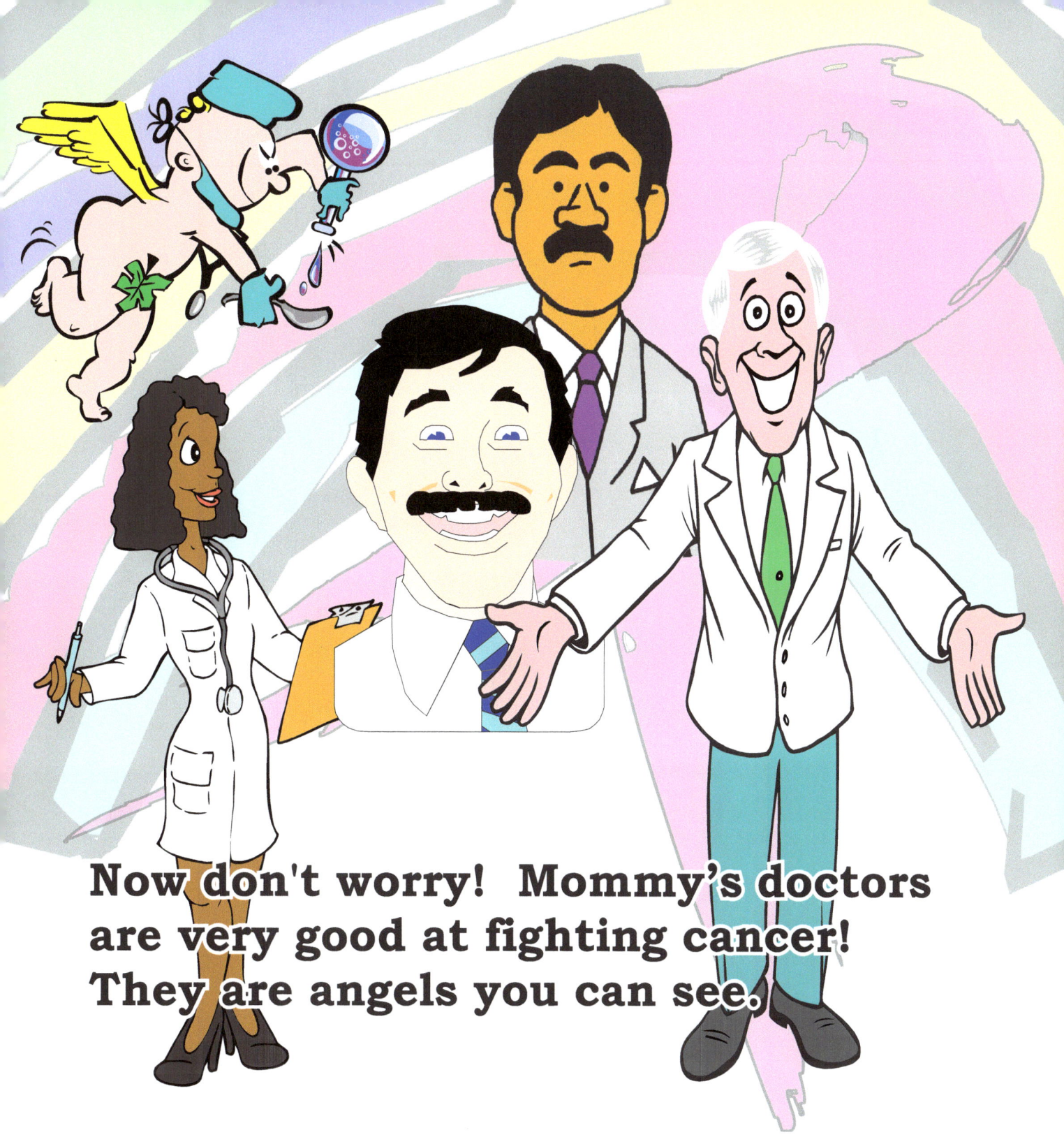

Now don't worry! Mommy's doctors are very good at fighting cancer! They are angels you can see.

All Mommy's doctors work together! It is like Mommy has her very own football team. All the doctors put their heads together and make a plan. The good cells win the game when Mommy is all better. YEAH TEAM!.

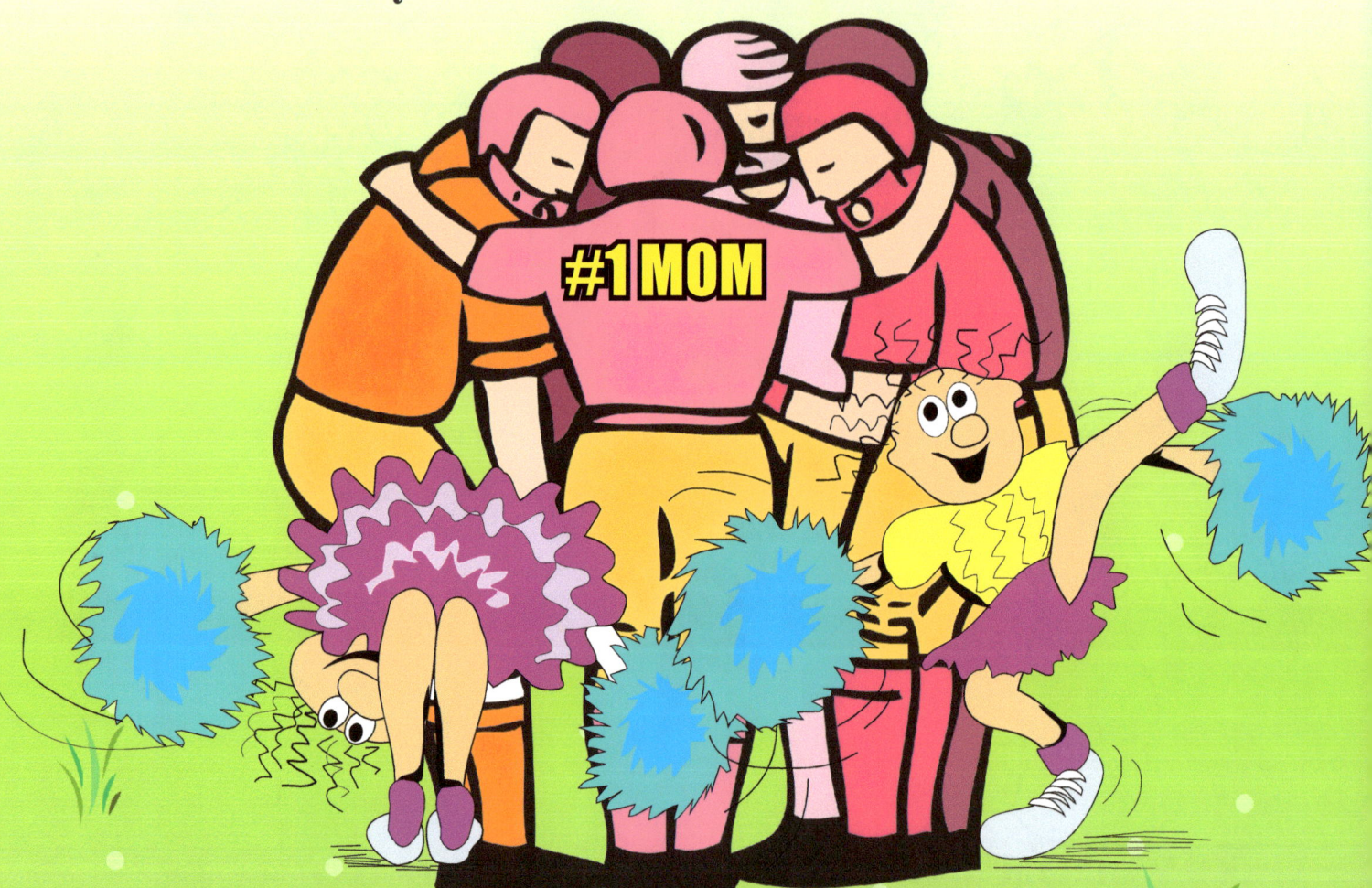

Mommy will still be her family's cheerleader, but for awhile she will have to cheer for you sitting down. Fighting cancer takes lots of energy. Always remember your love makes Mommy very strong!

Some days you may feel sad because Mommy is feeling sick... it's ok.

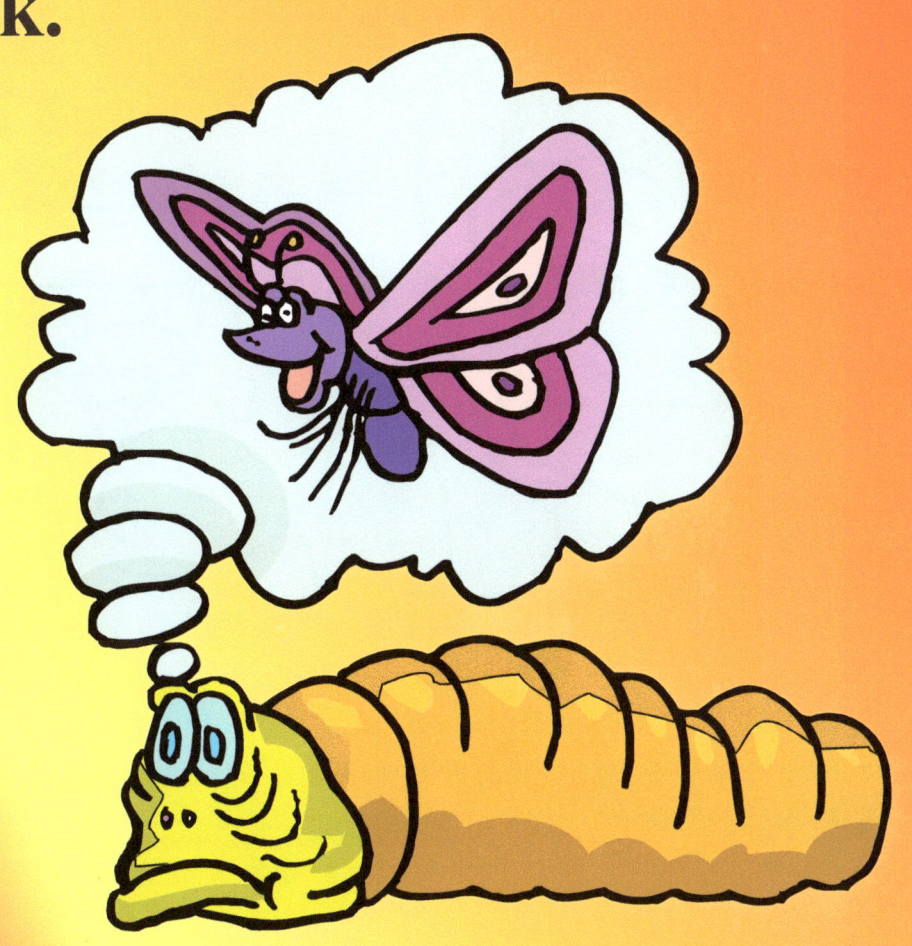

Some days Mommy just can't do all the things she used to do.

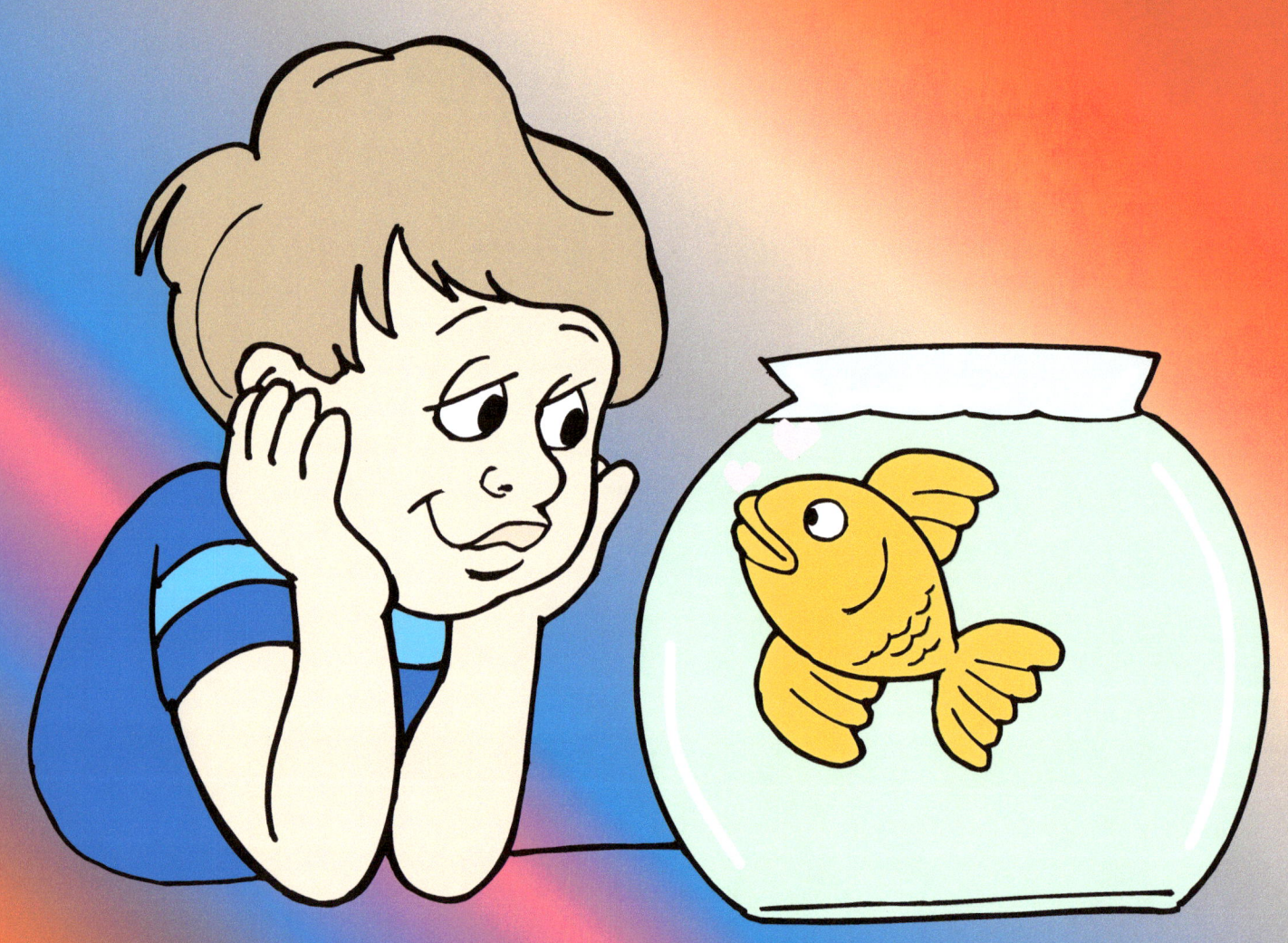

If you feel afraid you can talk to someone. It always makes people feel better to talk about their feelings.

Just say a prayer.

Children's prayers are music to God's ears.

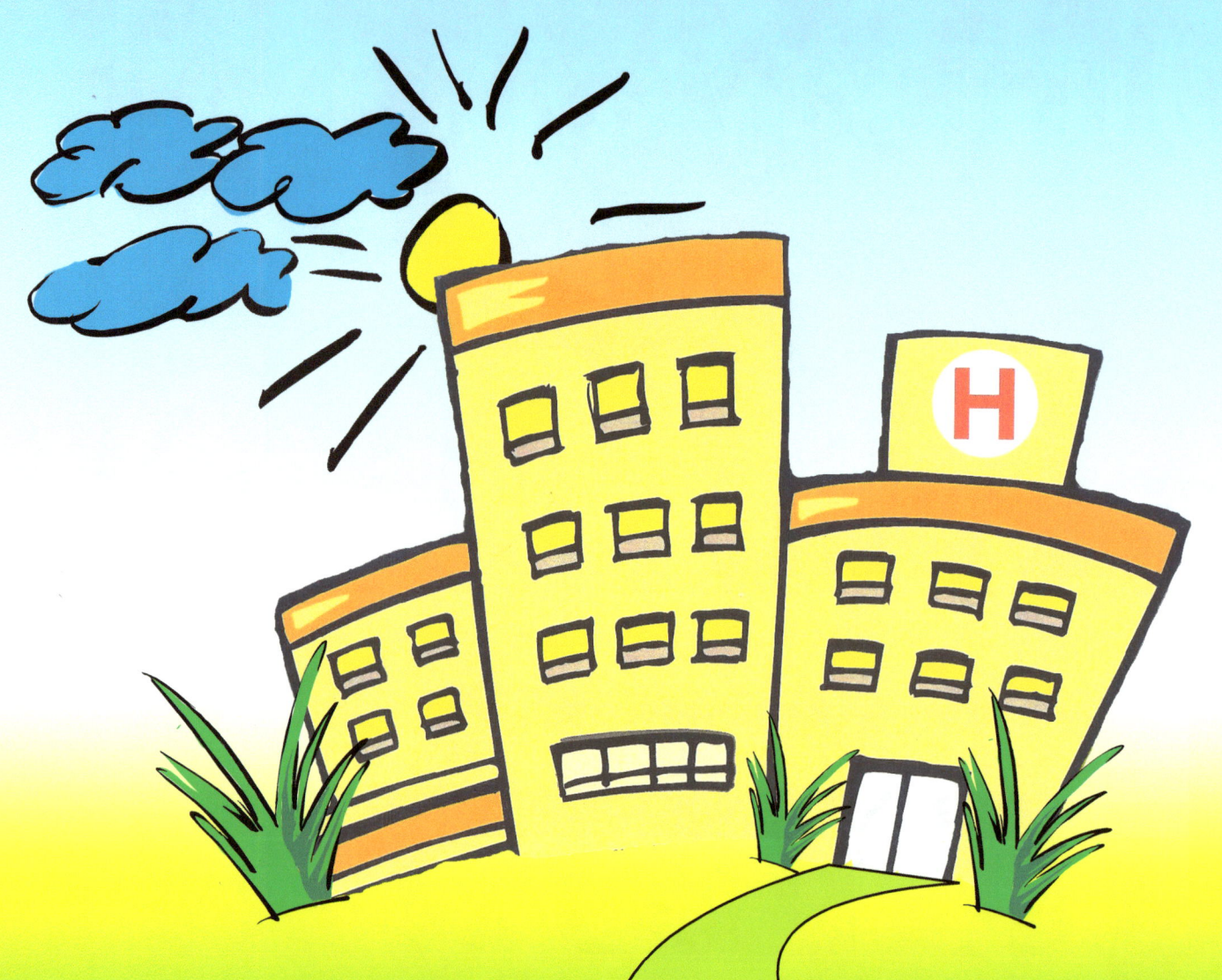

Mommy will do a couple different things to get better. Some will hurt a little bit and others will not hurt at all.

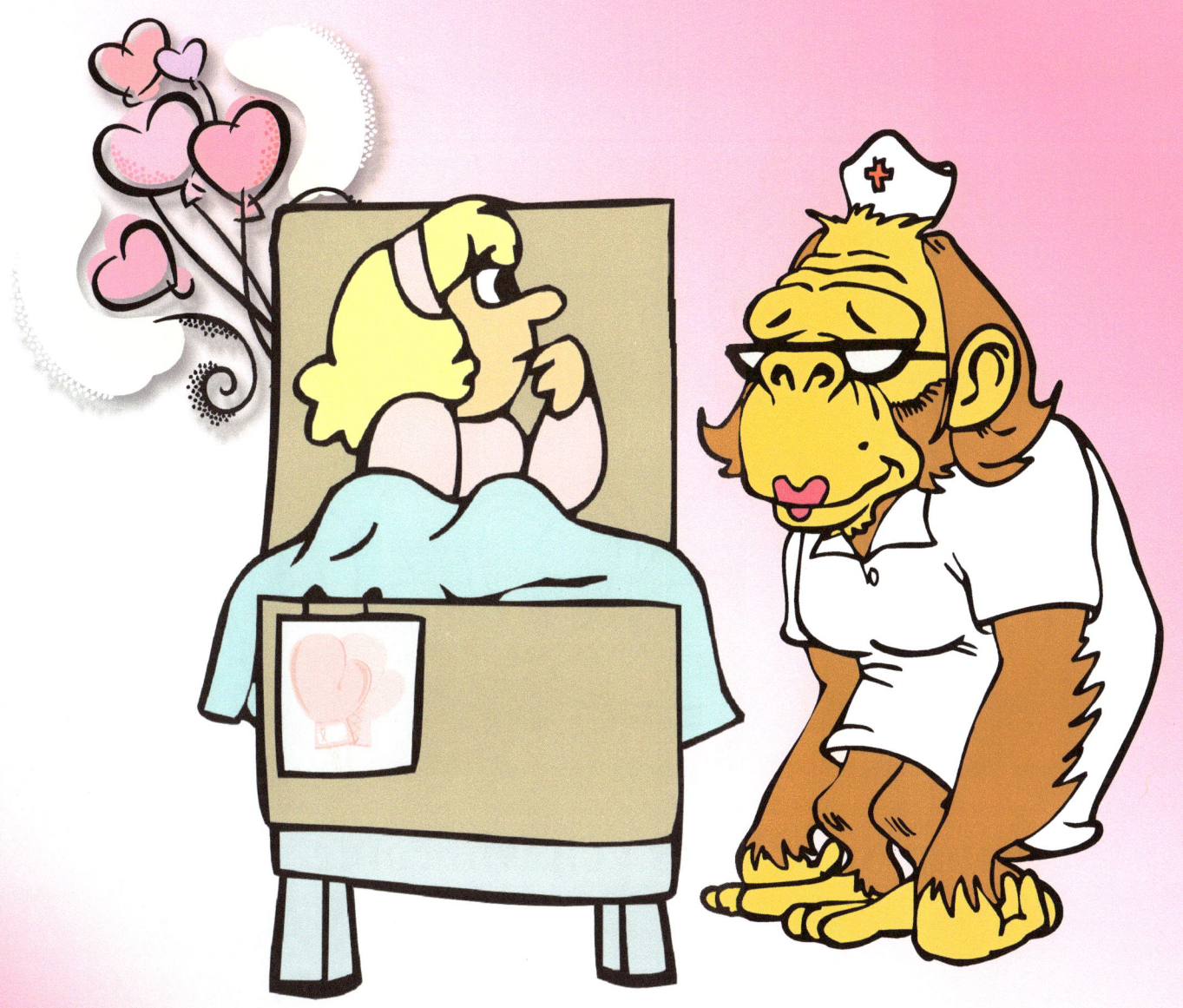

The first thing she will do is have surgery. She may be in the hospital for a few days. The doctor will take out Mommy's bad cells while she is sound asleep. She will not feel a thing and someone she loves will be right by her side when she wakes up.

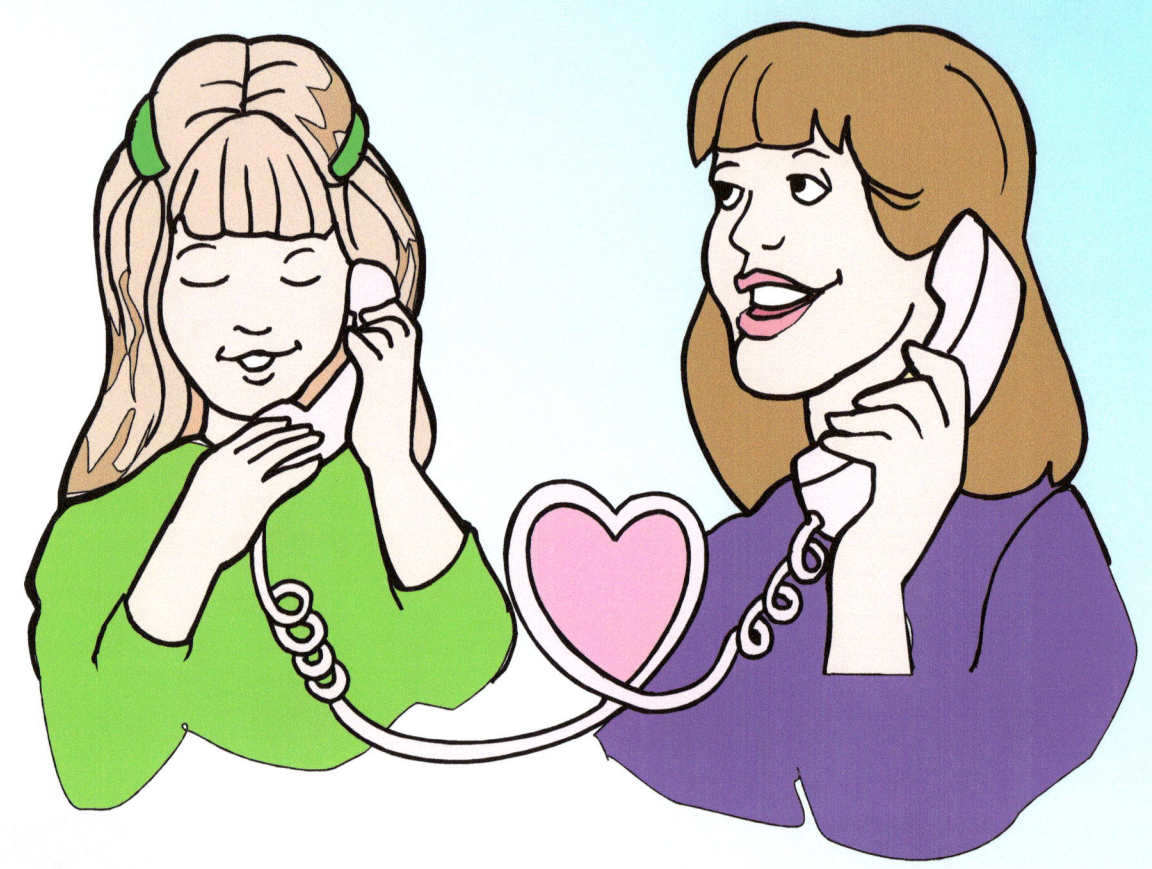

Someone who loves you will come and stay with you. Mommy will call every day to make sure that they are not spoiling you too much. If you miss Mommy, you can write her a letter or draw her a pretty picture. Mommy is never far away because she is always in your heart.

Next, Mommy may need something called RADIATION. The doctor will lay her on a table and put a strong beam of light over her chest and heat up the bad cancer cells. This helps to get rid of the bad cells. POOF!

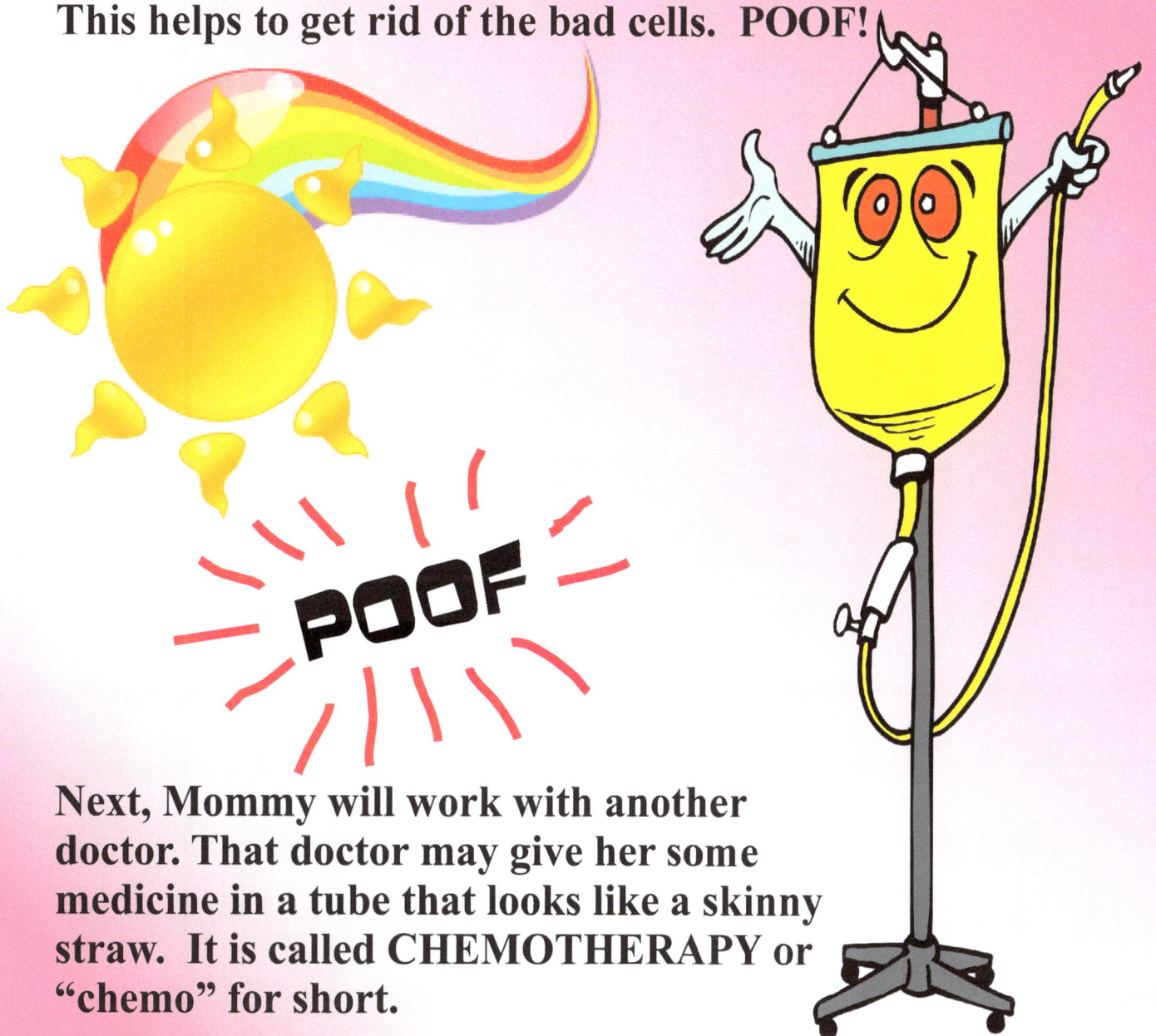

Next, Mommy will work with another doctor. That doctor may give her some medicine in a tube that looks like a skinny straw. It is called CHEMOTHERAPY or "chemo" for short.

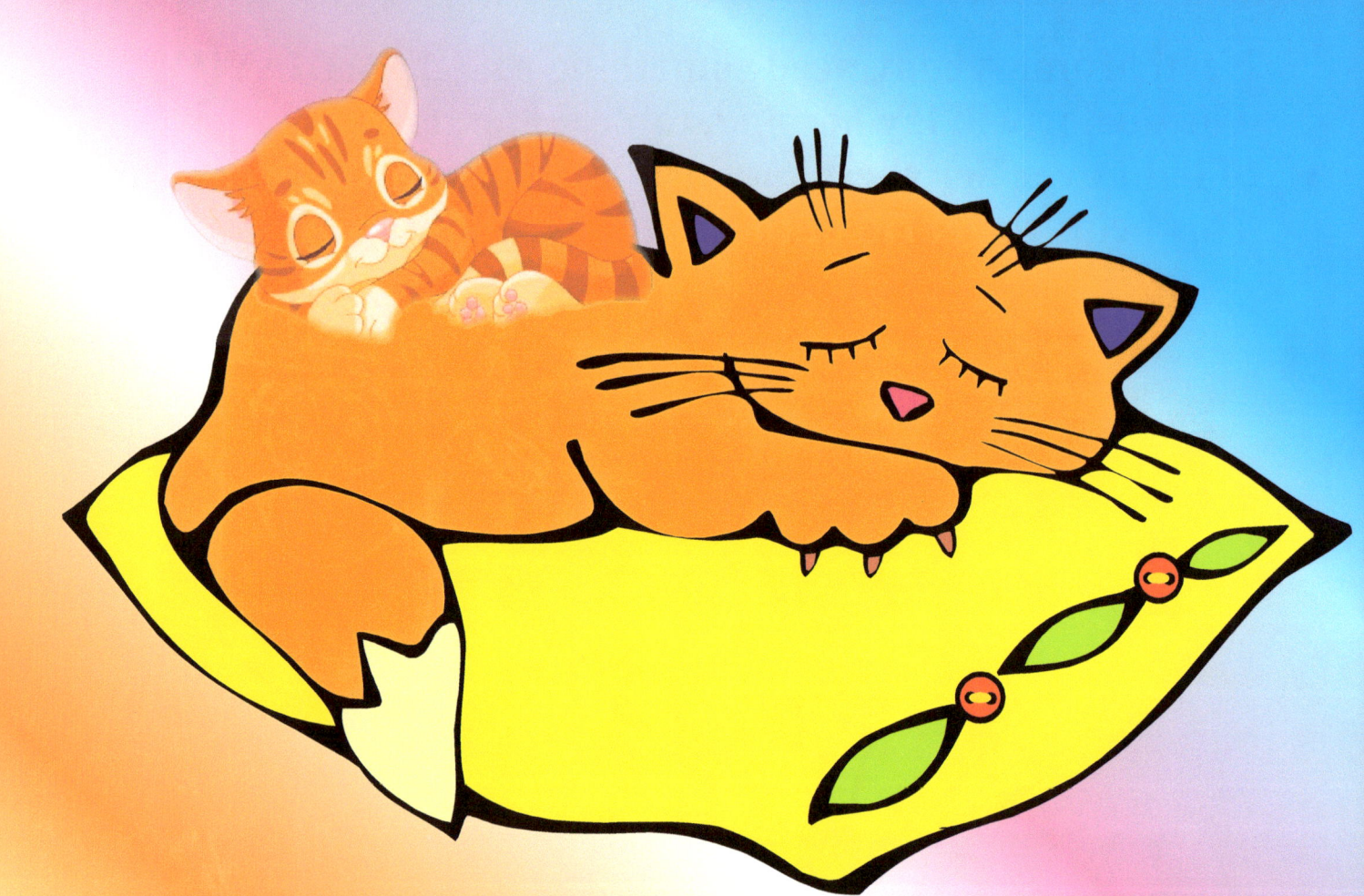

Chemotherapy will cause a few things to happen. Mommy will be very tired. She may even start to take naps like you did when you were little. You and Mommy can take naps together.

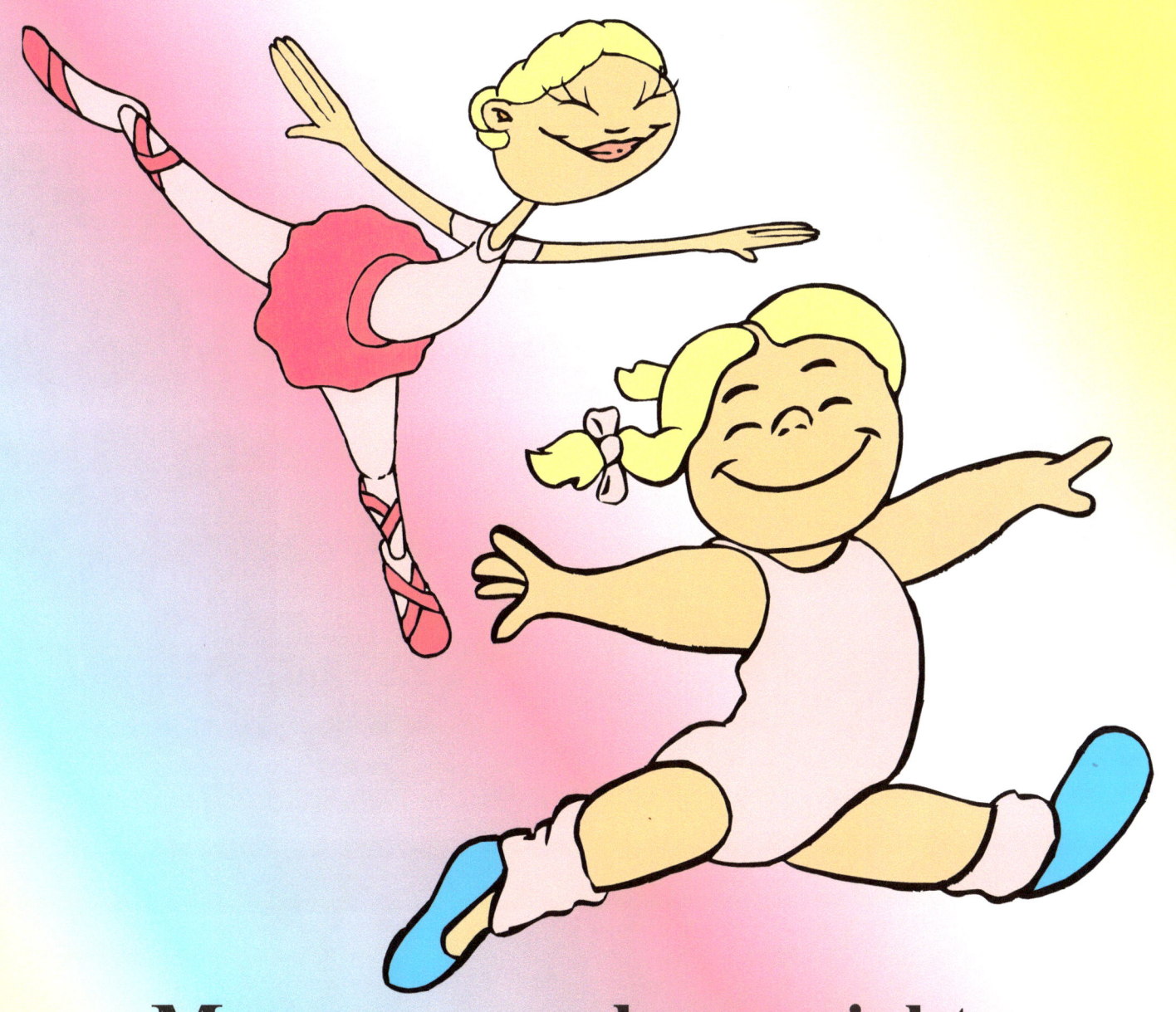

Mommy may lose weight or gain weight and it's ok.

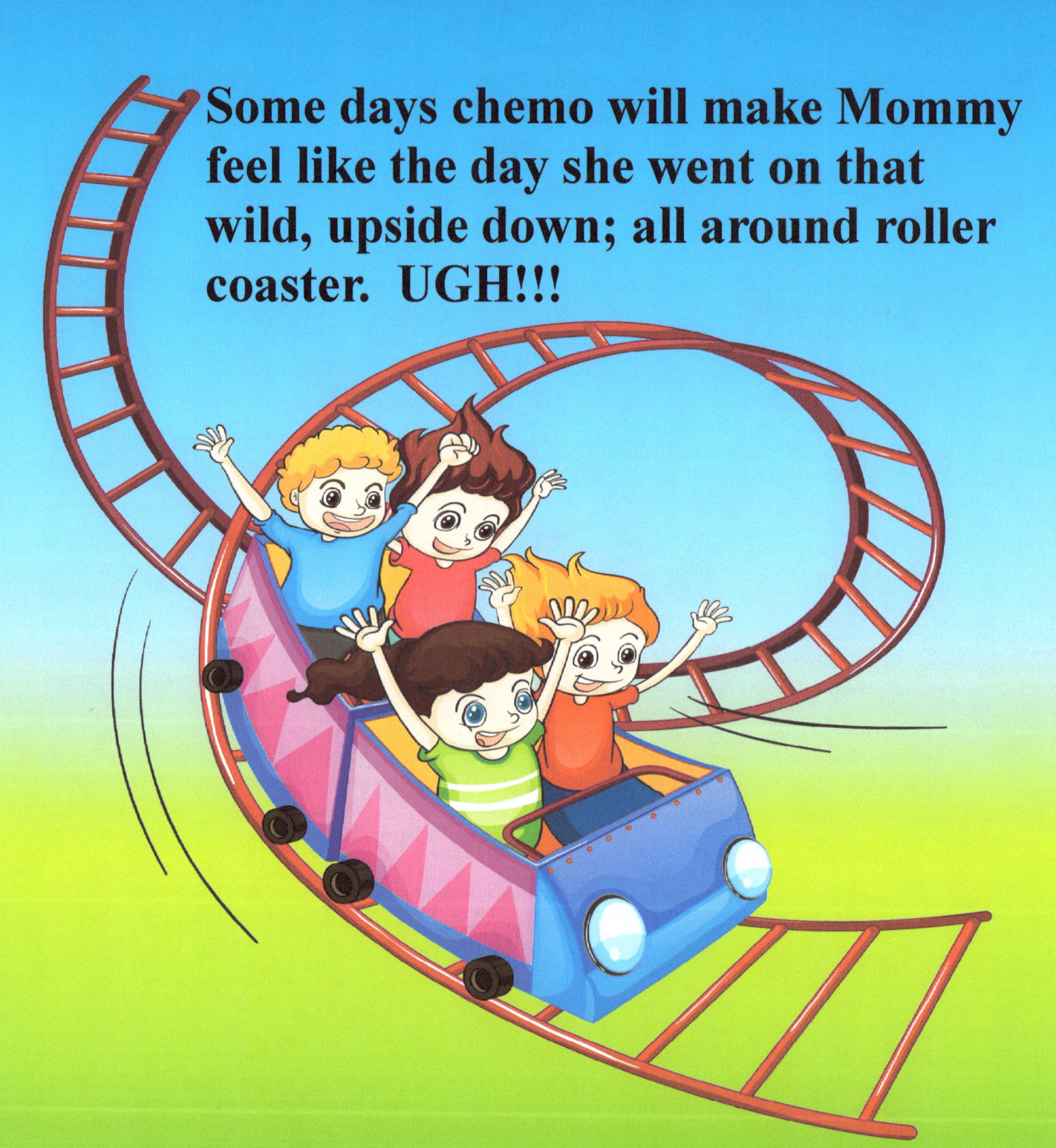
Some days chemo will make Mommy feel like the day she went on that wild, upside down; all around roller coaster. UGH!!!

On days when Mommy feels too sick maybe one of her friends will come to the house to cook and clean...

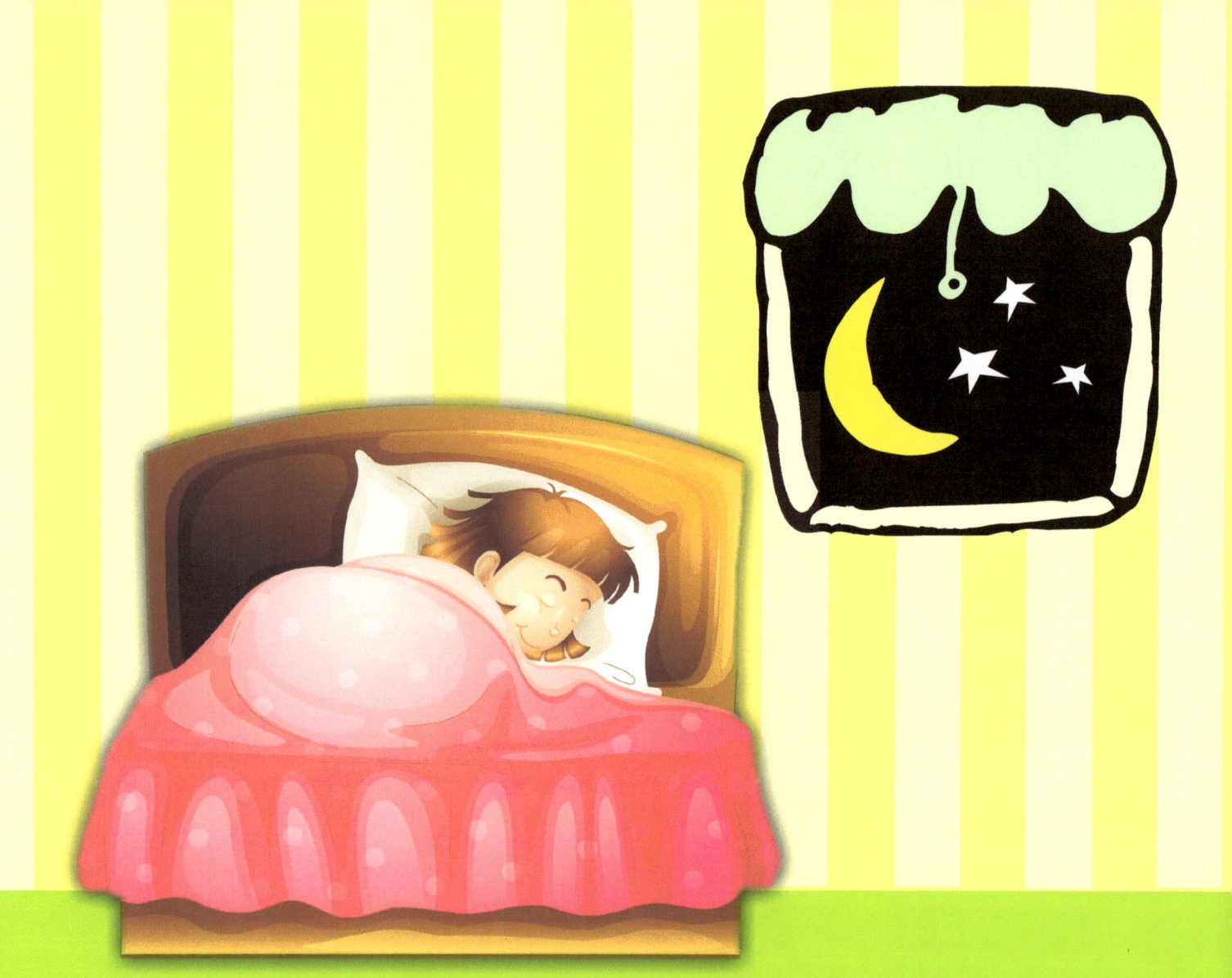

maybe even tuck you in at night. Mommy will always have the energy for goodnight kisses. Some nights you can tuck her in bed!

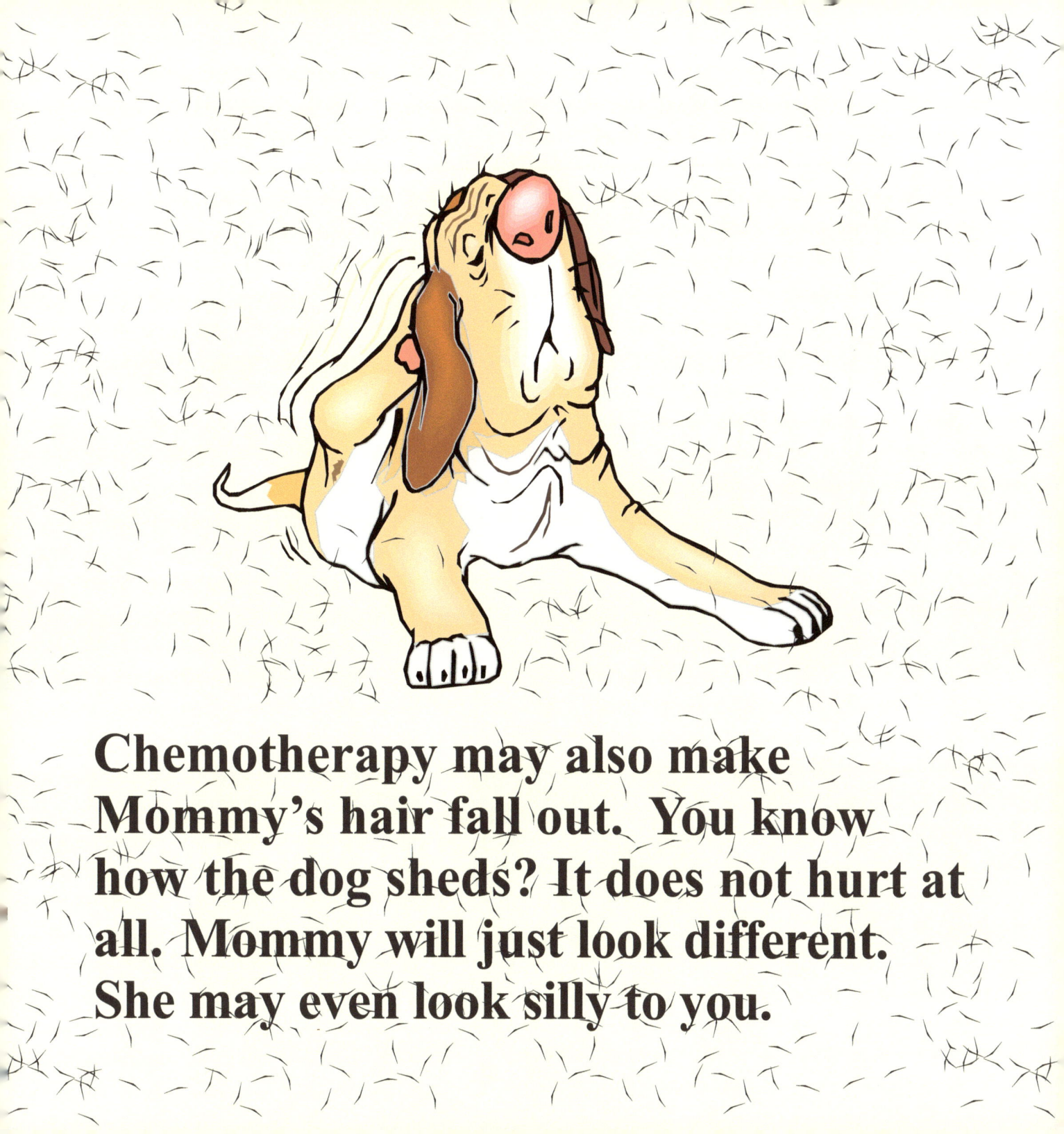

Chemotherapy may also make Mommy's hair fall out. You know how the dog sheds? It does not hurt at all. Mommy will just look different. She may even look silly to you.

Mommy will wear lots of pretty hats and scarves to cover up her bald head. Mommy may even wear a wig if she has someplace fancy to go.

Let's just hope it is not a very windy day!

Chemo is like winter when all the trees lose their leaves. In the spring all the leaves come back a bright green. The flowers bloom and spread their sweet smell.

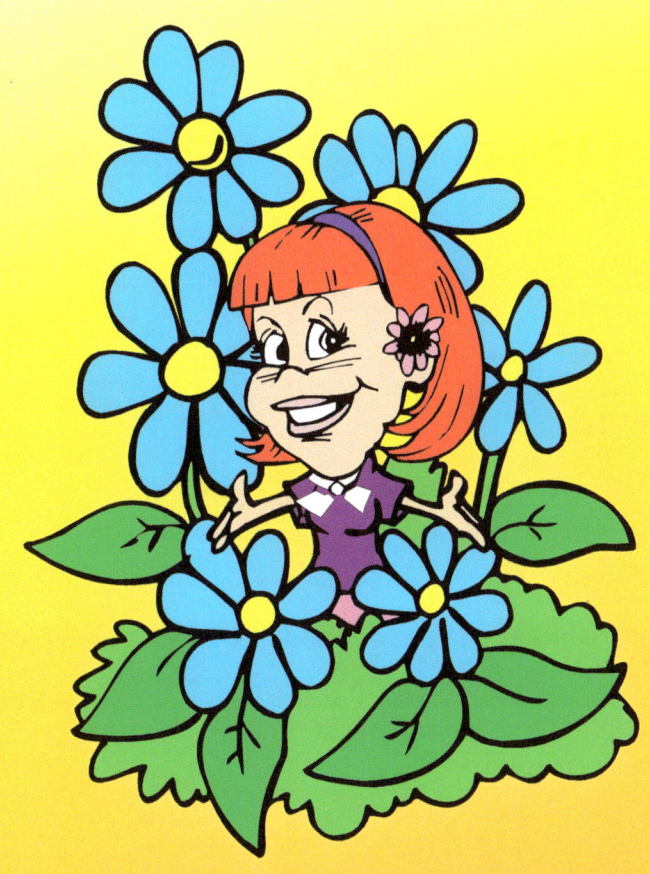

After chemo MOMMY will BLOOM AGAIN!

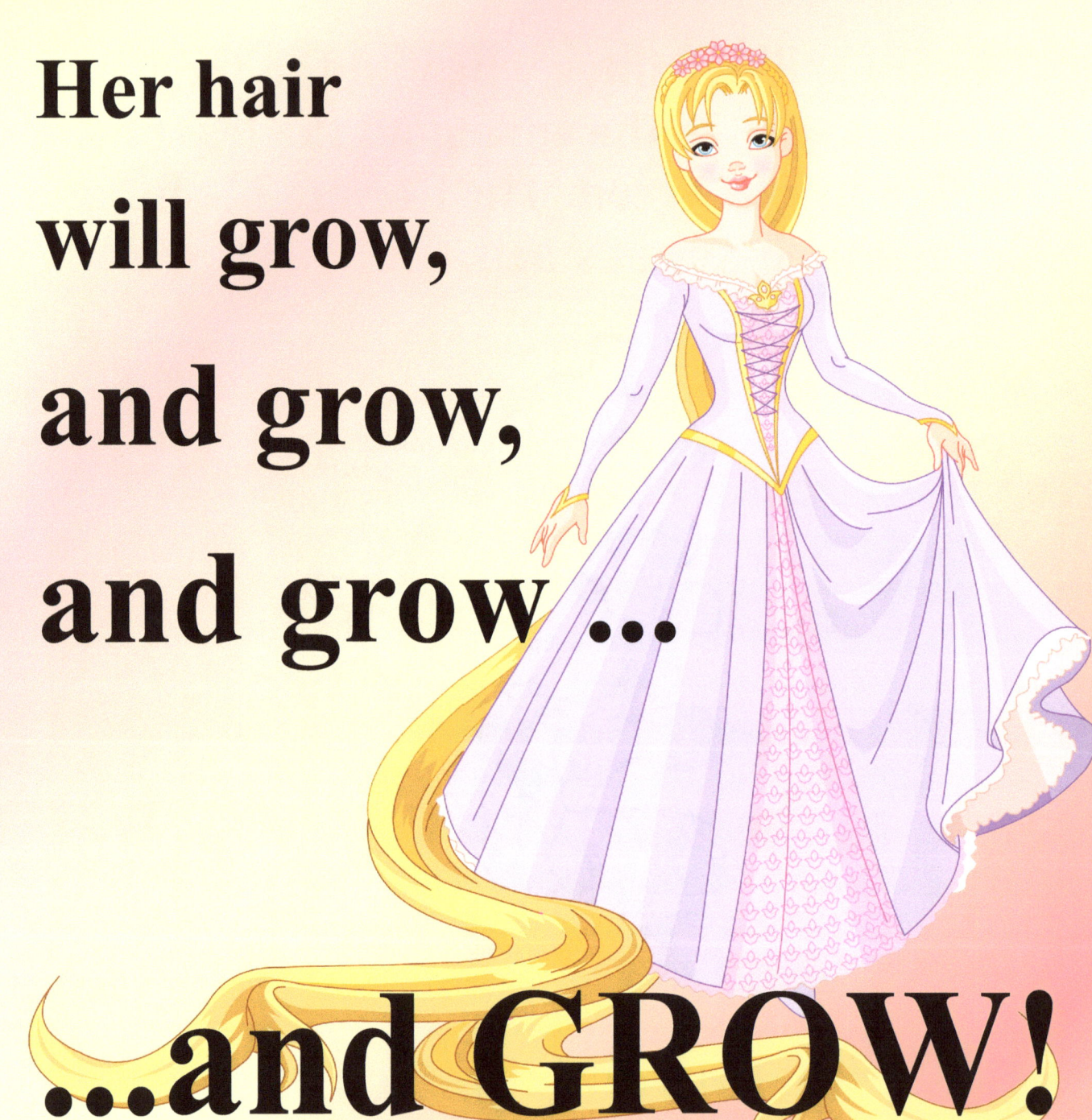

Her hair will grow, and grow, and grow ...

...and GROW!

Mommy will be radiant with... new health, new hair, and even a new outfit!

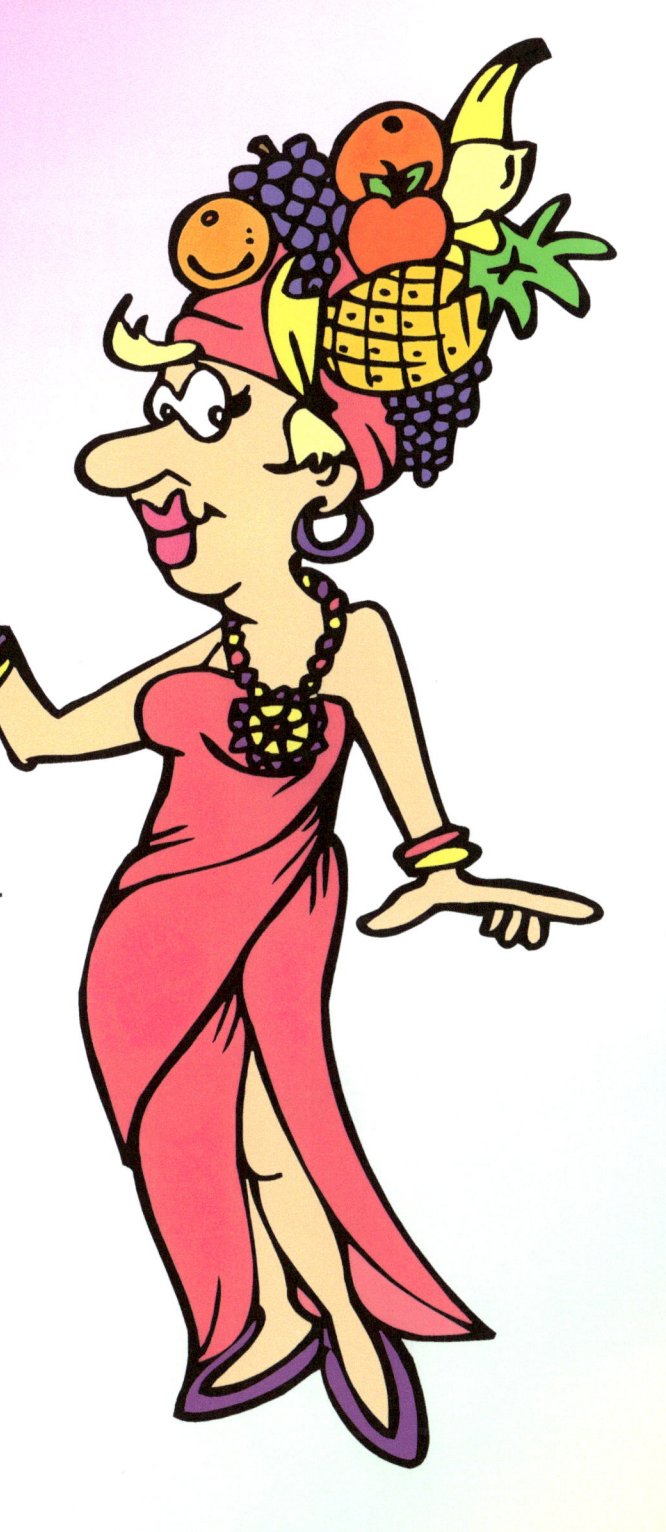

Our family will thank God for helping us climb this big breast cancer mountain.

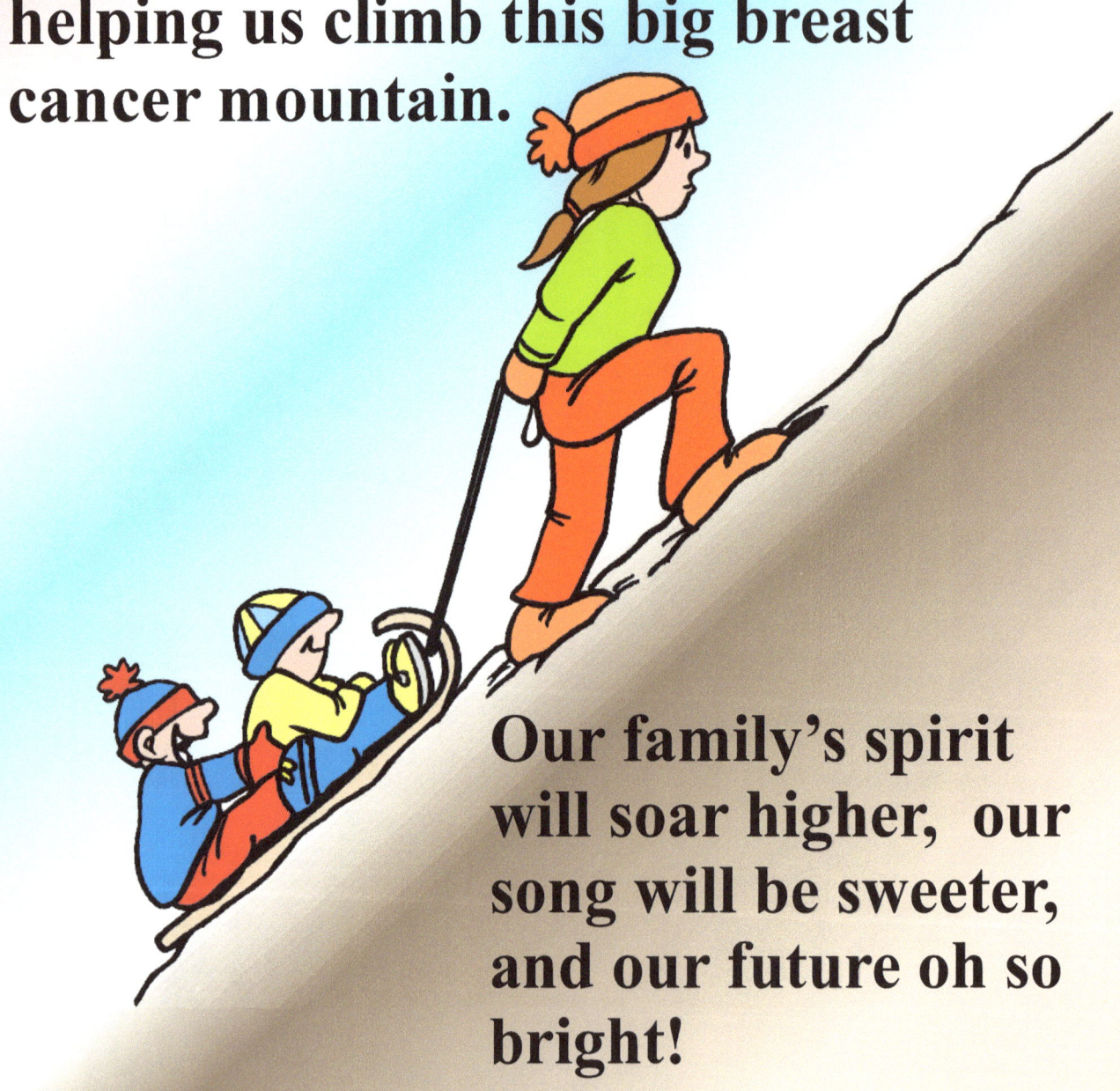

Our family's spirit will soar higher, our song will be sweeter, and our future oh so bright!

Cancer may change the way Mommy looks, but she is still the same loving Mommy inside.

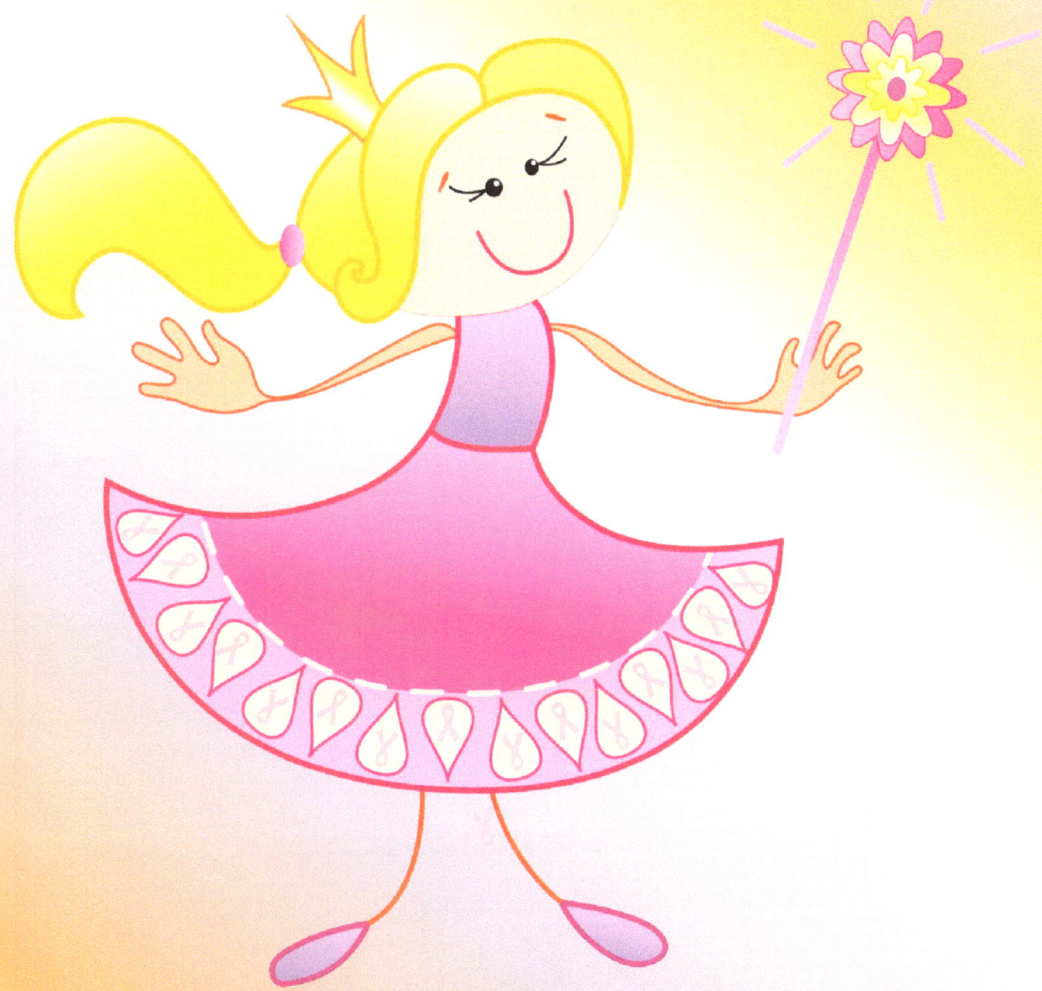

Her heart is the same, it is full of LOVE. Her eyes are the same, they dance when she sees you. Her smile is the same, it could light up the world when we are together.

Breast cancer..
can never stop the love of a Mommy.
A Mommy's Love Is ...

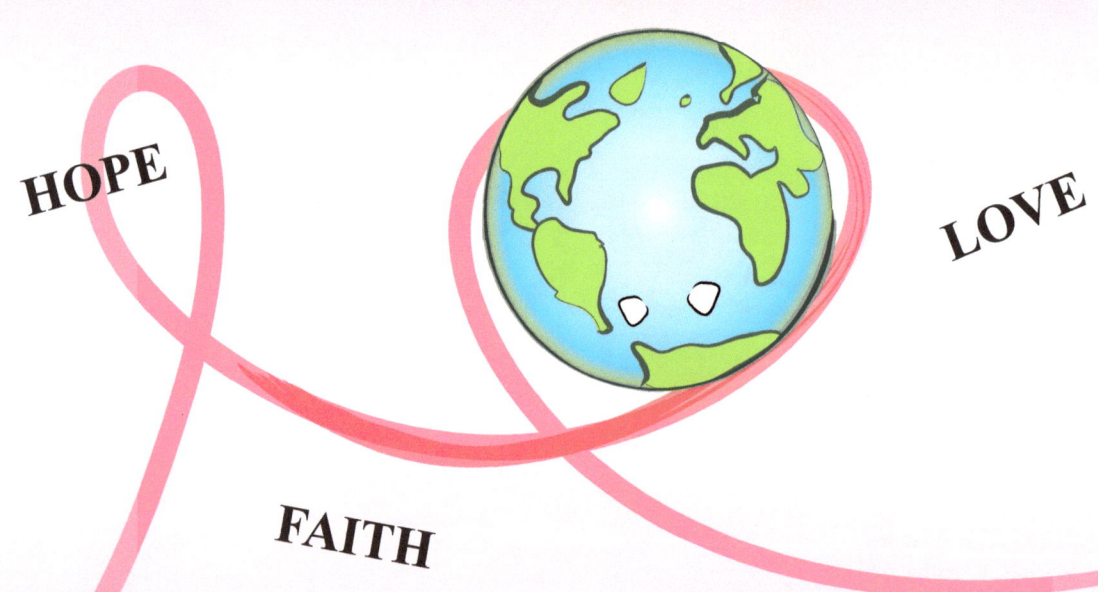

HOPE

LOVE

FAITH

Up to the Sky,
Around the World &
Deep in My Heart...

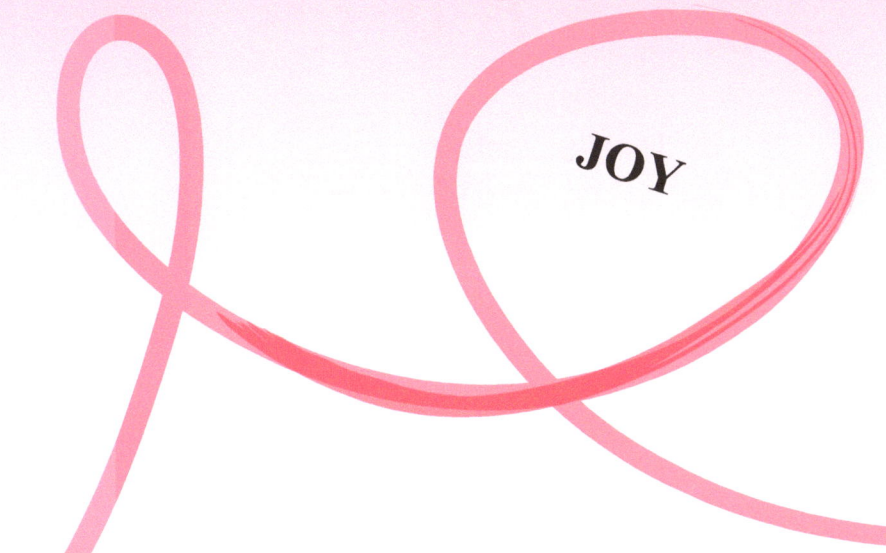

PEACE

JOY

FOREVER.

Up to the Sky, Around the World & Deep in My Heart

by Janelle Basham
illustrated by Kimberly Slingerland

A warm, hopeful and inspiring children's book to help children understand a mother's journey with breast cancer.

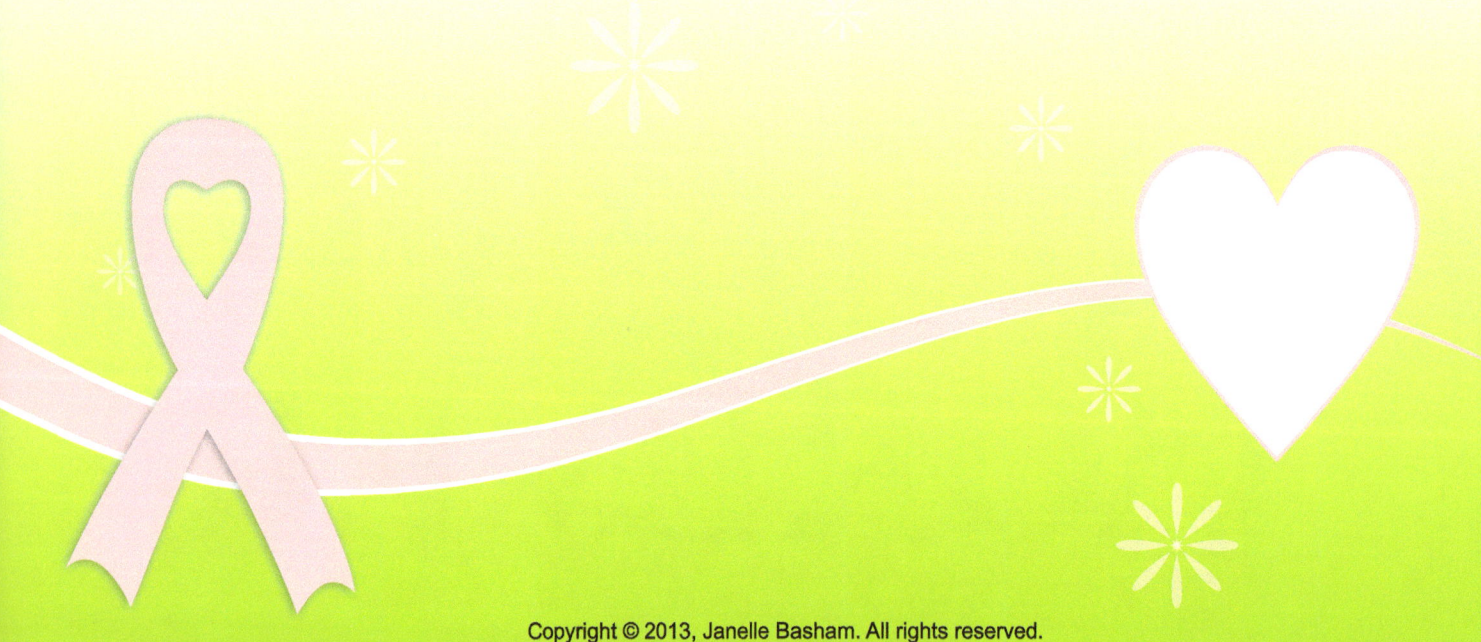

Copyright © 2013, Janelle Basham. All rights reserved.
Printed in the United States of America.

Congratulations
On your GREAT BIG Accomplishment

Name: _____

Message: _____

_____

_____

Congratulations you have completed this book successfully

Congratulations
On your GREAT BIG Accomplishment

Name: _____

Message: _____

_____

_____

Congratulations you have completed this book successfully

Congratulations
On your GREAT BIG Accomplishment

Name: _____

Message: _____

_____

_____

Congratulations you have completed this book successfully

Congratulations
On your GREAT BIG Accomplishment

Name: _____

Message: _____

_____

_____

Congratulations you have completed this book successfully

Congratulations
On your GREAT BIG Accomplishment

Name: _____

Message: _____

_____

_____

Congratulations you have completed this book successfully

Congratulations
On your GREAT BIG Accomplishment

Name: _____

Message: _____

_____

_____

Congratulations you have completed this book successfully